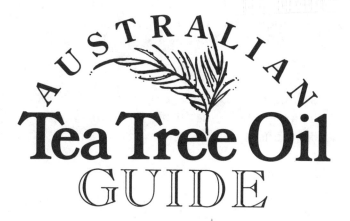

AUSTRALIAN
Tea Tree Oil
GUIDE

BY CYNTHIA B. OLSEN

PUBLISHED BY KALI PRESS

Second edition, Australian Tea Tree Oil Guide,
Copyright © 1991, 1989 by Cynthia B. Olsen

Edited by: Christopher S. Gerlach
Designed by: Kathy Reed
Typeset by: D G Associates
Published by: Kali Press, Fountain Hills, AZ

The author does not imply any medical solutions other
than the documented medical data that has been
provided. Consultation with medical people should
always be taken into consideration before treatment.

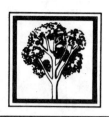

TABLE OF CONTENTS

"As we walk life's path there are always going to be the unexpected bumps, cuts, stings, burns, etc. For me, I can breath a little easier knowing that I have a bottle of Tea Tree Oil in my medicine cabinet—it is truly one of Mother Nature's bountiful gifts to man—it works, it works, it works."

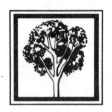

Introduction

I n the spring of 1986, I was introduced to a remarkable essential oil. While paying a call at a friend's house in Dallas, Texas, I was invited outside to visit the vegetable garden. While gazing at the plentiful fruits and vegetables my friend had grown with such loving care, I suddenly experienced a hot, burning pain on one of my legs. I jumped back and discovered I had been standing in a bed of fire ants. My friend rushed me to the house and, opening his medicine cabinet, produced a small bottle. While uncapping it, he proudly turned to me and exclaimed, "This will take the stinging and redness away immediately. This is a remarkable oil I discovered while living in Hawaii and it's a miracle oil. It's called Australian Tea Tree Oil."

Having been a student of natural medicine for twenty years, I had never come across Tea Tree Oil before. My friend was eagerly waiting to apply it to my injured leg. Being a hospitable guest and not wanting to appear rude, I allowed him to apply the Tea Tree Oil. If it would take the stinging away, I would gladly be a guinea pig. Within a minute of the oil being rubbed on my leg, all the pain and redness disappeared like magic. Thus began my introduction to Tea Tree Oil, an amazing first aid in a bottle that is just being discovered worldwide.

The Tea Tree, or Melaleuca alternifolia, grows naturally only in one region of the world: in the northeast corner of Australia. It is a full size tree, of the myrtle family, whose oil has powerful abilities to clean and help heal wounds and skin ailments in people and animals. It is one of the unique plants found in Australia.

Australia has many species of animals that are not found in any other part of the world. The funnelweb spider is found only in New South Wales, Australia where the Melaleuca alternifolia tree grows. The funnelweb spider is extremely toxic and a bite from the spider can cause death quickly. Since 1927, there have been seven reported deaths due to a bite from a funnelweb spider. I would like to quote from an account that occurred in May of 1983 from a Harry Bungwahl who resides in New South Wales:

"A rather extraordinary episode happened to me recently involving Tea Tree Oil. I was bitten on the foot by a funnelweb spider. It happened at nighttime about 1:00 a.m. He gave me a vicious bite and it was very painful. I lay down on the bed and tried to think of some way to soothe the pain of the bite which was very severe. I then thought of the small bottle of Tea Tree Oil which was in the bathroom. My wife went and got it and applied some to the bite and there was an immediate easing of the pain. My wife then went to ring up Taree Hospital and while she was doing that, I put some more Tea Tree Oil onto the bite, which in a short time stopped being painful! My son drove me to the Taree Hospital. The foot was no longer painful, but my lips and fingers were still tingling. The spider was identified as a male funnelweb spider alright. I was given no treatment, but was kept under observation for a period of four hours and then discharged."

My purpose in writing this guide is to share with people who are looking for alternative medicines the wonderful story of the Australian Tea Tree Oil. My wish for you is that your family, your friends and your pets will be able to experience Tea Tree Oil and have it in your medicine cabinet. Once you use it, you'll wonder how you ever got along without it, believe me. So, let's begin the amazing story of the Australian Tea Tree Oil, otherwise known as Melaleuca alternifolia.

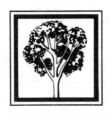

Acknowledgements

I wish to extend my thanks to the following people who contributed to the guide:

Christopher Dean, Governing Director of Thursday Plantation, Ballina, N,.S.W., Australia. Chris provided much of the clinical data. Also, his sincere efforts to bring Australian Tea Tree Oil to the world marketplace should be recognized here.

The photographs were provided by Terry and Eve O'Leary of Main Camp, Casino, N.S.W.

Thanks to the N.S.W. Tourism Commission, Los Angeles, California. Rick Matkowski helped to locate an accurate map of the N.S.W. region.

The Australian Trade Commission, Los Angeles, California. Jim McNicol was willing to answer a myriad of questions.

Finally, a sincere thank you to Robert Cook who introduced me to Tea Tree Oil five years ago.

From the Land of Wonder

An estimated sixty million years ago, as the continents of earth continued to shift and change shape, an immense landmass measuring more than three million square miles gradually separated from the Asian mainland and formed the largest island on earth—*Australia*.

"The Lucky Country," "The Quiet Continent," "Last of Lands," "New Australia," and "New Holland" are just a few of the names used by seventeenth-century Dutch explorers to describe this island of contradictions. It is a land that has been called "upside down," because, unlike the United States or Europe, southern Australia faces toward Antarctica and is relatively cool. By contrast, the northern region is near the equator, warm and tropical, and supports a rich diversity of life ranging from the mountains to the plains, vast deserts of the outback to peaceful lagoons, lush rain forests to the Great Barrier Reef.

Foremost among the rare and unusual trees growing along Australia's northeast coast, in the swampy, low-lying lands of New South Wales, is the Melaleuca alternifolia or "Tea Tree."

"...We at first made it <some beer> of a decoction of the spruce leaves; but finding that this alone made the beer too astringent, we afterwards mixed it with an equal quantity of the tea plant (a name it obtained in my former voyage from our using it as tea then, as we also did now) which partly destroyed the astringency of the other, and made the beer exceedingly palatable, and esteemed by everyone on board."

Captain Cook's account of his second voyage, A Voyage Towards the South Pole (Vol. 1, p. 99, 1977)

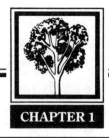

CHAPTER 1

History of Australian Tea Tree Oil

Captain Cook Discovers the Extraordinary Tea Tree

I n 1770, Captain James Cook (at that time a lieutenant) of the British Royal Navy landed from the H.M.S. Endeavor at Botany Bay, near the eventual site of Sydney. From there the party continued their way up through the northeastern coastal region (now New South Wales) where they came upon groves of trees, thick with sticky, aromatic leaves that, when boiled, rendered a spicy tea. A botanist with the expedition, Sir Joseph Banks, collected samples of the leaves and brought them back to England for further study. These early explorers could not have known that 150 years later, Melaleuca alternifolia, or "Tea Trees" as they were called by Captain Cook, would be used as a medicinal agent for cuts, burns, bites, and a host of skin ailments.

Penfold Study

In 1923 an Australian curator and chemist at the Government Museum of Technology and Applied Sciences in Sydney, Dr. A.R. Penfold, conducted a study of the leaves of the "Tea Tree" and discovered their essential oils to be thirteen times stronger as an antiseptic bactericide than carbolic acid, considered the universal standard in the early 1900's. In 1925 Penfold announced his findings before the Royal Society of New South Wales and England.

"Melaleuca alternifolia is quite common, and exists in very large areas in the North Coast district of New South Wales. It yields 1.8% of an oil of pale lemon tint, with a pleasant terpenic myristic odor. This is prepared on a commercial scale, and is particularly recommended as a non-poisonous non-irritant antiseptic and disinfectant of unusual strength, the Rideal-Walker coefficient being 11. The oil contains 50-60% of Terpenes (pinene, terpinene and cymene), from 6-8% of Cineol (accounting for the camphoraceous odor) and an alcohol terpineol, which supplies the pleasant nutmeg-like odor, also small amounts of sesquiterpenes and their corresponding alcohols....The valuable antiseptic properties of the oil and its spicy flavoring note should prove useful in dentifrices and mouthwashes."

Pre-World War II

Research continued, and by 1930 the editors of the Medical Journal of Australia reported that applying the Tea Tree Oil to pus-filled infections dissolved the pus and left the surface of infected wounds clean and without apparent irritation to the healthy tissues. The article also stated that application of Tea Tree Oil on infected nail beds eradicated the damage within one week. It was also noted that a few drops of oil, in a tumbler of warm water as a gargle, helped to soothe sore throats. In 1933, journals such as the *Australian Journal of Pharmacy, The Journal of the National Medical Association (U.S.A.)* and the *British Medical Journal*, stated that "the oil is a powerful disinfectant, non-poisonous and non-irritating, and has been used successfully in a very wide range of septic conditions." Research indicated that Tea Tree Oil was successfully administered around the world for throat and mouth conditions, for gynecological conditions, and in dental treatment for pyorrhea and gingivitis. It also had an extraordinary effect on a variety of skin fungi including candida, tinea and perionychia. Even before World War II there were scientific claims being established about this unique oil. In 1936, *The Medical Journal of Australia* reported that Tea Tree Oil successfully treated diabetic gangrene. Also, in 1936 a magazine called *Poultry* announced that Tea Tree Oil (known at that time as Ti-Trol) prevented cannibalism in poultry. When the Ti-Trol was applied to chickens, the odor of the oil kept the chickens from pecking at one another. In 1937 it was noted that in the presence of blood, pus, and other matter, the oil's antiseptic features were increased 10-12%.

World War II

During World War II, Tea Tree Oil was considered to be such a necessary commodity that cutters and producers were exempted from war service until sufficient reserves of the oil had been accumulated to permit its standard issue in first aid kits for the Army and Naval units in the tropical regions. Large quantities of Melaleuca alternifolia oil were blended with machine cutting oils, to kill bacteria, and reduce infections from skin injuries, especially abrasions to the hands by metal filings and turnings. Eventually demand exceeded supply and synthetic alternatives were developed.

Synthetic drugs gained popularity as miracle drugs and eventually pushed Tea Tree Oil into the shadows. But with the arrival of the 1960's and "flower power," a new awareness took hold throughout the West. Toxic substances and synthetic medicine began to lose favor as a new generation turned to natural medicines. By the 1970's, Tea Tree Oil was rediscovered.

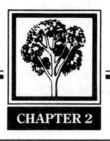

CHAPTER 2

Harvesting and Production

Tea Tree Oil Composition

The Melaleuca alternifolia (MA) is made up of forty-eight unique organic compounds, some of which have never been found in nature, so names had to be created. One of these compounds is called viridflorene. It appears that all forty-eight unique compounds work in synergy to produce an essential oil that has antiseptic and fungicidal properties. The oil color may vary from colorless to pale yellow. The aroma is pungent and resembles eucalyptus. The bush oil appears to have a heartier aroma than plantation oil.

Two of the chemical compounds that are tested from batch to batch are cineole and terpinen 4-ol. Both of these ingredients need to meet certain percentages according to the Australian standard. (Refer to the standard at the end of this chapter.) If cineole is above 15%, it will become caustic to the skin. In reality, cineole should be 5% or less. Terpinen 4-ol should be above 30%; in fact, the higher the better, since this compound contains healing properties.

Even though Tea Trees have been studied since 1923, there is much more to be discovered about them. For instance, the trees grow in a specific region of New South Wales and yet the oil, upon testing, may vary from batch to batch and tree to tree. Even the tried and true old method of steam distilling the oil may affect and change the consistency of the compounds.

Tea Trees have not always been looked upon as a wonder of

nature. In fact, for years Australian farmers considered them a nuisance. The farmers desired to clear the trees off their land so they could raise cattle. Tea Trees have tenacious root systems that go deep. Yanking out a tree is not an easy task and if any roots are left intact, the tree will surface again quickly.

Bush Oil

The natural habitat of Melaleuca alternifolia is the swampy, low-lying land around Clarence and Richmond River systems where a multitude of established trees thrive. (See map in Chapter Two.) There are over three hundred varieties of Melaleuca; however only one, the Melaleuca alternifolia, contains great amounts of antiseptic and fungicidal qualities.

Currently, the only area where Melaleuca grows in its natural state is in the northern region of New South Wales. The consistency of the oil varies from tree to tree. However, the trees that grow in the Clarence-Richmond River areas appear to contain higher levels of terpinen-4 ol and lower levels of cineole, which produce an ideal combination for healing purposes.

For many years, a score of small producers would venture into the area with skilled leaf cutters and prepare to harvest the branches of the trees. The Melaleuca alternifolia, a narrow-leafed paper bark tree twenty feet in height, thrives in remote "flood-prone" wetlands; therefore, harvesting the leaves is extremely laborious. The cutters use light-weight, razor-sharp machetes to cut the suckers off the stumps before stripping each branch with a cane knife. The dense bush has prevented all attempts at mechanized harvesting where even four-wheel drive vehicles frequently get trapped in the mud.

In spite of these obstacles, experienced cutters work very quickly and are able to cut one metric ton of leaves in a day using a simple technique of holding branches upside down with one hand while cutting with the other. This method of harvesting prevents any damage to the trees or the surrounding eco-system.

In fact, the growth of the tree seems to be stimulated by regular cropping. Some of the trees along the Bungawalbyn Creek have been harvested for over sixty years and are most healthy and hardy. Experienced cutters can harvest a ton of leaves in a day's work, which yields ten liters of oil.

Once the leaves are pruned, they are brought to a steam distiller unit also called a "bush still." The still is heated by wood and the harvested leaf is placed on racks inside the steamer. Once the water boils to a certain temperature, the steam passes through the leaves. The capillaries burst, releasing the essential oil where it passes to a collection tank. The oil floats to the top where it is filtered and then poured into containers to be shipped to various marketplaces.

Plantations

Most of the production of the oil has been derived from the natural stands of trees. However, there are pitfalls that occur with the production of bush oil. Besides being labor-intensive due to the inaccessibility of the trees, production is limited and adverse weather can affect the operation.

With the increasing interest in Tea Tree Oil, the growers and producers are beginning to plan ahead so that supply will be able to keep up with world-wide demand. Thus, Tea Tree plantations started appearing in the mid 80's and are now springing up all around New South Wales. Although operating costs are high, the agricultural system is efficient to keep production costs down.

The season for production of the oil is in the Australian summer, which is December through May. The trees grow rapidly during the hot summers and appear to slow down their growth in the winter months. If frost occurs, growth will stop.

Since Tea Trees require rain, plantations have had to rely on irrigation. Tea Trees tolerate flooding, although full immersion may kill trees if they are flooded for more than a week.

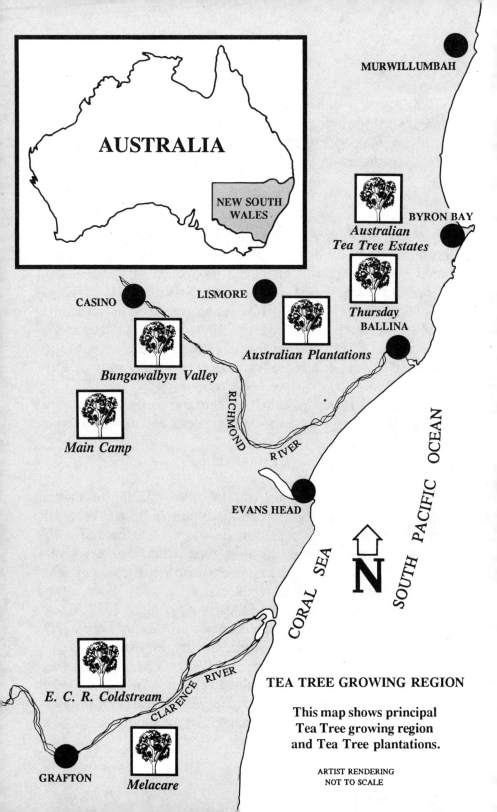

AUSTRALIA

NEW SOUTH WALES

MURWILLUMBAH

Australian Tea Tree Estates

BYRON BAY

CASINO

LISMORE

Thursday
BALLINA

Australian Plantations

Bungawalbyn Valley

RICHMOND RIVER

Main Camp

EVANS HEAD

CORAL SEA

N

SOUTH PACIFIC OCEAN

E. C. R. Coldstream

CLARENCE RIVER

TEA TREE GROWING REGION

This map shows principal
Tea Tree growing region
and Tea Tree plantations.

GRAFTON

Melacare

ARTIST RENDERING
NOT TO SCALE

Soil that is composed of sandy loam or light-textured soil appears to be preferable for growing Tea Trees. Planting in valleys with good irrigation is important as well. Wind drys the limbs, so sheltering the plant helps to reduce damage.

Transplants

Since Tea Tree seeds are extremely small, it is more economical to establish seedlings in trays. Collecting seeds from good quality trees will affect the production of the plantation. Seeds can be collected year-round. Seeds mature in 12—18 months. Seedlings take 7—10 days to germinate in the summer months. Once the seedlings are 10—15 cm. tall, they can be transplanted. Transplanted seedlings can produce thirty to forty thousand plants per hectare (equivalent to slightly over an acre). Yields of 150—200 kg. per hectare can result.

The plantations establish a nutrition system which may include fertilizing the plants. Weeds, pests and diseases also are observed.

Production

The annual production of Tea Tree Oil in the eighties amounted to 15—20 tons. With more plantations appearing, the production has now increased to sixty tons. That number could conceivably rise to seven hundred tons within the next several years. There is also increasing interest from foreign countries to purchase the oil in bulk amounts.

The Australian Tea Tree Industry Association (A.T.T.I.A.) was formed to establish guidelines for the industry. The members are made up of growers, buyers and exporters.

Given the increased interest in the Tea Tree industry, there is a strong indication that it could develop into an industry worth $20—$25 million within the next ten years. The price of the oil also may fluctuate due to the changes in the supply and demand of the product.

Due to the increased awareness in the world marketplace for Melaleuca alternifolia, the temptation is great (and at the moment unfortunately "allowed," following the current standard) to dilute Melaleuca alternifolia oil with other oils and to use a Tea Tree Oil that is not from Melaleuca alternifolia. No clinical data has been produced to support the efficacy of a blended oil. Since Tea Tree compounds are so unique, blending other types of Tea Trees (over 300 varieties) or blending other types of oils may affect the careful balance that nature has provided. More studies will need to be put into effect to make that determination. Accept only authentic Melaleuca alternifolia oil.

Hence, it is important for distributors and the consumer to be certain that the Tea Tree Oil they sell or use is authentic antiseptic grade Tea Tree Oil that falls into the guidelines of the Australian Standard. The following table shows the acceptable Australian standard:

Australian Tea Tree Oil Standard

Australian Tea Tree Oil is mentioned in the British Pharmaceutical Codex of 1949, Martindale's listing of Australian Approved Names, the U.K. Medicine List, and the Dispensary of the U.S.

There is an Australian standard for Melaleuca alternifolia, that being AS 2783-1985, superseding the former standard (AS 175-1967). The current standard permits blending of other Tea Tree Oils while assuring that the terpinen-4 ol content is at least 30% with 15% cineole.

The old standard was specifically for Melaleuca alternifolia and clearly designates Melaleuca alternifolia as being the oil for therapeutic uses.

This requirement to use only Melaleuca alternifolia is now regarded by the Australian Tea Tree Industry Association [ATTIA] as essential.

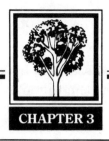

CHAPTER 3

Medical Research

Pena Study: Yeast Infections

I n the late 1950's and early 1960's, Dr. Eduardo F. Pena, M.D. investigated Melaleuca alternifolia oil for effectiveness in eradicating both trichomonal vaginitis and candida albicans. A further purpose of this study was to observe any possible irritation or side effects and to determine the proper strength of the oil for safety and efficacy. The solution consisted of an emulsified 40% solution of Australian Melaleuca alternifolia oil with 13% isopropyl alcohol. This special emulsion results in the solution being miscible with water in all proportions, giving a milky appearance when diluted.

The study was conducted on 130 women suffering from four types of vaginal infections: 96 cases of trichomonal vaginitis, several cases of thrush and cervicitis, and a control group of 50 women who were treated with anti-trichoma suppositories. Out of 130 patients, all treatment was successful and the Tea Tree Oil treatments had similar results to the control group. In the 96 cases of trichomonal vaginitis, clinical cures were obtained by inserting a tampon saturated with a 1% solution of Melaleuca alternifolia oil which was then removed after twenty-four hours. Daily vaginal douches of 1% solution in one quart of water were also recommended. The number of office treatments necessary to achieve a clinical cure averaged six, while the total number of douches per patient averaged forty-two. Patients commented of its pine odor and its soothing, cooling effect. It was also apparent that at no time did the patient experience irritation or burning. **The clinical study indicated that Tea Tree Oil is a penetrating germicide and fungicide with additional characteristics of dissolving pus and debris.**

M. Walker Foot Problems, April, 1972

In a study done on various foot problems, i.e.: athletes foot, fungal infections, under-toenail corns, and callouses, Dr. Walker used Tea Tree Oil in three different formulas. First as a pure oil; second 40% oil with 13% isopropyl alcohol (which allows the oil to be water miscible—giving it another name, Melasol) and thirdly; 8% oil with lanolin and chlorophyll. Sixty patients were involved in the study. Forty were put on Melasol, twenty applied the ointment and eight used the pure oil. Treatments varied from three weeks to four years. Out of sixty-eight patients, fifty-eight found relief from their foot problems over a period of six years. At least four different fungal conditions are affiliated with athletes foot, all of which responded well using Tea Tree Oil.

Belaiche, First Study:
Thrush (Candida Albicans)—September, 1985

Dr. Paul Belaiche, Chief of Phytotherapy Department at the Faculty of Medicine, University of Paris, has worked on several studies involving Tea Tree Oil. One study was conducted on patients with thrush, a vaginal infection of candida albicans. Although there are usually low levels of candida albicans normally found in the vagina, the growth is kept under control by certain bacteria. It is when an increasing amount of antibiotic treatment is used that the healthy bacteria ceases to flourish and the candida albicans proliferates. Some indications of infection are itching, white discharge and pain. Dr. Belaiche's study focused on twenty-eight patients using a Tea Tree Oil suppository inserted into the vagina every evening. One week later, one patient discontinued treatment due to vaginal burning. Thirty days later upon examination, twenty-one out of twenty-eight patients showed a complete recovery. The remaining seven were clinically, but not biologically cured. Dr. Belaiche felt Tea Tree Oil to be very effective, less irritating than other essential oils, and easily tolerated by vaginal membranes. **"The essential oil of Melaleuca has entered the team of major essential oils and emerges as an antiseptic and anti-fungal weapon of the first order in phyto-aromatherapy."**

Belaiche: Second Study, Chronic Cystitis

Twenty-six female patients, with an average age of thirty-nine, were given a capsule of Tea Tree Oil once a day over a three-month period. Because this was a double-blind study, two lots of thirteen patients each were formed. Lot A was given twenty-four mgs. of Melaleuca alternifolia daily—three doses of eight mgs. before main meals. Lot B received a placebo. After six months, Lot B showed no improvement, while in Lot A, seven (out of thirteen) were cured.

In addition to these findings, Tea Tree Oil was found to be effective on staphylococcus, streptococcus and candida albicans. It was shown to be equally effective on other skin disorders such as acne and impetigo. Perhaps the most impressive results were studies of fungal nailbed infections: eight out of eleven patients recovered using two applications per day, with a treatment time of one to three months.

Acne Study Done by Lederle Laboratories
and Royal Prince Alfred Hospital, Fall 1990
Benzoyl Peroxide Versus Tea Tree Oil

An acne study was completed in the fall of 1990 comparing benzoyl peroxide water based lotion with a Tea Tree Oil gel containing 5% Tea Tree. Five of the 124 patients that participated did not complete the study because they had been on antibiotics for treatment of other illnesses. Sixty-one people were in the benzoyl group and fifty-eight in the Tea Tree group. No topical acne treatment was used two weeks prior to the trial study.

Due to the difference in color and aroma between the two acne treatments, the three month study was conducted as a single blind study; the investigator being "blind." Also, none of the patients were aware of which treatment they were receiving.

The study showed a 5% Tea Tree Oil gel was effective as a topical acne treatment; due to the slower onset of action, it was less effective than the benzoyl lotion. Benzoyl's action was probably due to established properties as a keratolytic agent, which Tea Tree Oil probably does not have.

Although the Tea Tree solution was slower acting, greater dryness was experienced by 79% of the benzoyl group versus 44% in the Tea Tree group after one month's time. Tea Tree Oil was also better tolerated by facial skin.

Since the Tea Tree Oil gel was administered at only 5% solution, another study may be done using higher concentrations of the oil. Acne has been treated successfully using 100% Tea Tree Oil in the past, according to anecdotal reports.

The acne study was a first as far as the use of Tea Tree Oil being compared to a common pharmaceutical preparation in a clinically controlled trial. Also, having a major pharmaceutical company conducting the test is important to note here.

Tea Tree Oil Study

Tea Tree Oil was tested recently in 1991 in a family practice office. Fifty patients with various skin problems were chosen at random. The purpose was to test and confirm the efficacy and safety of using high quality Tea Tree Oil. Several varieties of the oil were used including the pure oil (100%); lozenges with 1% oil and some of the ground leaf, and a cream (5%). All products were supplied by Thursday Plantation, Ballina, N.S.W., Australia. Thursday Plantation was one of the pioneers of the revival of the Tea Tree industry.

The fifty patients tested consisted of eighteen men, thirty women and two children, ages ranging from four to ninety-three. The treatment lasted from one to four weeks depending on the severity of the condition to be treated. One patient dropped out of the study and a second discontinued due to a mild erythematous skin sensitivity to the 100% oil. This was the only side-effect reported.

The results of using the Tea Tree Oil were striking. All the patients but one were cured or showed remarkable improvement of the conditions treated. The single case of eczema resistant to the oil had the pruritus decreased.

Dr. Alvin Shemash and Dr. William Mayo feel that further studies should be made on athlete's foot, tinea versicolor, seborrheic, dermatosis, psoriasis, hemorrhoids, vaginal moniliasis, chicken pox and herpes zoster rashes.

The doctors also noted that Tea Tree Oil is a natural, less costly, effective alternative to drugs with fewer side effects.

The following table summarizes the conditions that were treated:

Condition	No. of Patients	Product Used
Mild facial & back acne	8	Cream
Monilia of throat/mouth	13	Lozenges
Monilial rashes of skin	6	Cream
Non-specific dermatitis, eczema	4	Oil/Cream
Infected pustules	1	Oil
Oral canker sores	3	Oil
Herpes simplex-face & lips	6	Oil
Fungus of fingernails, tinea cruris, pedis & barbae	7	Oil/Cream
Total Patients	48	

Tea Tree Oil Use for Bacterial Vaginosis and Monilial Vulvovaginitis

Bacterial vaginosis—A patient having been diagnosed with bacterial vaginosis refused a pharmaceutical drug (metronidazole) and instead used Tea Tree Oil pessaries which contained 200 mg. of Tea Tree Oil. The treatment lasted five days and a one-month followup showed the condition cleared. Tea Tree Oil may be a safe, non-toxic alternative to standard antibiotic therapy as noted by Dr. Blackwell, *(Lancet, December 8, 1989)*.

Monilial vulvovaginitis—Dr. Donald Brown has treated female patients having them use the pessaries every other day for a total of six treatments—extended to twelve if necessary. These are patients that have not responded to nystatin pessaries, for instance. Dr. Brown has used a 15% solution of Tea Tree Oil on acne vulgaris as well.

Geriatric Test
Podiatry Training Clinic, Sydney, Australia

Another recent study completed at Royal North Shore Hospital used a Tea Tree Oil hand and body lotion containing a 5% solution of Tea Tree Oil. The purpose of the study was to compare the legs of people who were diabetic and geriatric in nature. The seventy people suffered from dry skin and/or debilitating diseases such as diabetes.

The patients were asked to use the cream only on one leg for a period of 25-26 days. A marked difference was noticed on the leg that received the cream. Dry skin became much softer, cracks healed and disappeared. Tea Tree Oil's potential as a bactericide and skin emollient was noted. This study is important due to the ages of the people and their having fragile and thinner skin which may be easily damaged and take longer to heal.

American Society
for Environmental Education

11 July, 1989

Cynthia Olsen Teaco
P O Box 389
SANTA BARBARA   CALIFORNIA   93192
U.S.A.

Dear Cynthia,

I am writing you to tell you how very much I am personally
impressed with the Tea Tree Oil products from Australia.

My personal physician, Dr. Alvin Shemash has also been
quite pleased with results he has had with skin problems
with his patients after I introduced the product to him
recently.

I have found in my own personal experience that the Tea
Tree Oil is a fantastic curative for most any kind of
dermatological problems including nasal ulcer, athlete's
foot and rashes of all kinds.

My organisation the American Society for Environmental
Education has long had an interest in natural medicinal
products because of our overriding interest in the
environment and curative products occurring naturally. For
instance, we recently did some research on the medicinal
value of plants known to Indians in the Brazilian
rainforest, so you can see that the Tea Tree Oil fits right
in with our overall concern for the value of natural
products.

Please feel free to use this letter in your upcoming
publication on Tea Tree Oil or in any other way that you
may find it to be useful in heralding this fine natural
product.

Yours sincerely,

Williams L. Mayo Ph D
PRESIDENT

17

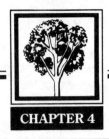

CHAPTER 4

First Aid Guide

Treatments for Nose, Sinus, Throat, and Chest Conditions

Blocked Nose/Sinus—Add ten drops of pure oil in steam bath vaporizer. Gently inhale.

Nasal Ulcers—Apply pure Tea Tree Oil with cotton bud or follow above treatment.

Sore Throat—Add five drops of pure oil to a cup of warm water and gargle two to three times a day.

Congestion/Coughs—Add ten drops pure oil to steam bath or vaporizer—inhale. Rub pure oil into chest and back. Sprinkle on pillow before sleeping.

Treatments for the Mouth

Sore Gums, Bad Breath, Plaque—Add three to five drops to water and use as a mouthwash twice daily. Add a few drops to toothbrush.

Mouth Ulcers/Cold Sores—Dab on pure oil three times per day.

Muscle and Joint Distress

Muscle Aches—Gently massage painful area. Rub pure oil into muscles. Add ten drops to hot bath and soak.
Arthritis—Mix three to five drops into a small amount of a quality cold-pressed oil such as almond oil.
Sprains—Rub pure oil into sprains for relief.

Treatments of Skin Ailments

Boils—Apply pure oil three times daily.
Cuts—Dab on pure Tea Tree Oil or mix one part Tea Tree Oil with ten parts of almond oil.
Abrasions—As above.
Dry Skin, Rashes—As above.

Mosquitos/Bites/Stings/Sandflies—Dab on pure oil. Apply Tea Tree and cold-pressed oil for large areas.
Leaches, Ticks—Apply pure oil to kill parasite, remove parasite and apply oil again.
Dermatitis—Massage oil into affected areas using 1 part Tea Tree to 10 parts other oil

After Shaving or Leg Waxing—Use a small amount of pure oil or Tea Tree lotion.
Pimples, Acne—Dab on three times per day or add three to six drops of pure oil to warm water and rinse affected area. Apply Tea Tree Cream for day-time treatment.

Minor Burns—Flush with cold water/ice pack immediately. Apply pure oil to burn. Apply Tea Tree Cream.

Sunburn—Apply Tea Tree Cream for immediate relief and to prevent blistering. For severe cases apply pure oil.
Tropical Ulcers, Plantar Warts, Coral Cuts—Dab on Tea Tree Oil three times per day.

Treatments for Foot Conditions

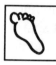 **Athlete's Foot**—A fungal condition that may be chronic or acute, often contracted in locker rooms. Sweating may also contribute to the condition. Wash feet with an anti-fungal soap and dry thoroughly. Apply pure Tea Tree Oil or Tea Tree Cream twice daily. A Tea Tree Oil soak may also prove beneficial. As suggested before, a solution of Tea Tree Oil and water may be used to disinfect areas and clothing.

 Nail Infections—Perionychia is a fungus of the fingernails and toenails. Often caused by synthetic nails or harsh detergents, the nail may become infected deep-down. Soak fingernails or toenails in pure Tea Tree Oil for five minutes, massaging the solution into the nailbed, twice daily until infection clears.

 Smelly Feet—Add five to ten drops of pure Tea Tree Oil to warm bath water, or rub oil directly into feet.
Carbuncles—Dab on pure oil twice per day.

Baby Care

 Diaper Rash/Change Lotion—Apply warm oil and lotion. *Do not use pure oil.*
Diaper Cleanser—Add twenty drops of pure Tea Tree Oil or a water miscible formula to each gallon of water. Stir and soak diapers overnight.
Cradle Cap—Use Tea Tree Oil Shampoo mixture, keeping away from eyes. Mix five drops of pure oil with olive oil, rub into scalp, leave for five minutes, then wash and rinse.

Treatments for Hair and Scalp

 Dry Hair—For those with dry hair that requires a kind, non-detergent based product a 2% solution of Tea Tree Oil in a moisturizing shampoo will help unblock sebaceous glands and encourage the free flow of the body's own moisturizing oils while clearing away unsightly dead skin cells. Shampoo daily or during usual routine and work up rich lather with a small amount of shampoo mixture. Rinse and shampoo again. Condition, if possible, with a 2% solution of Tea Tree Oil moisturizing conditioner.

Oily Hair—A gentle Tea Tree Oil moisturizing shampoo will help cleanse the scalp of bacterial and fungal irritations and help disperse dead skin cells. Shampoo daily. Using a few drops of Tea Tree Oil rubbed into the scalp will also aid dry scalp, oily scalp, itchy scalp, and dandruff.

 Head Lice—(Pediculus humans capitis). Headlice are common among school children and are often transmitted by combs, brushes, hats, bed linens, etc. Infestation normally occurs on the scalp. The headlice, appearing as small greyish white specks, bite and puncture the scalp causing pain and itching. The problem may persist due to the hatching of new eggs approximately every two weeks. Apply a Tea Tree Oil shampoo boosted with ten additional drops of pure Tea Tree Oil. Leave on ten minutes, then rise. Repeat procedure once or twice a week. Soaking combs, brushes, and other contaminated material in a Tea Tree Oil solution will also guard again continued infection.

Itchy Scalp—Use Tea Tree Oil shampoo or a few drops of Tea Tree Oil directly on scalp.

Pet Care

 Fleas—Wash using a few drops of oil in a pet shampoo, starting with the neck and working down the body. Repeat as required. Between shampoos, sponge 10-20 drops of pure oil into coat.

Rashes—Apply pure oil or Cream.

Cuts/Itches—Apply pure oil diluted, if required, with olive oil.

Suggested Formulas

1. One part of pure Tea Tree Oil with ten parts of a cold-pressed oil such as olive, apricot, almond, avocado, etc.
2. Add ten drops to an 8-ounce bottle of human shampoo.
3. Add ten drops to an 8-ounce bottle of pet shampoo.
4. Add ten drops to bath or humidifier, or vaporizer.

Precautions

1. Avoid contact with eyes.
2. **Do not store pure oil in plastics, as it may dissolve the container.**
3. Store in a cool place.
4. Keep out of reach of children.
5. Use of Tea Tree Oil should not be viewed as a substitute for professional medical care. If the problem persists, consult a doctor.

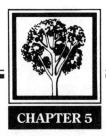

CHAPTER 5

Case Studies and Testimonials

Some Reports from Australian Practitioners

Re: **Mouthwash.**—"I advise five drops to four ounces of water which I consider quite strong enough for cleansing and germicidal results."

re: Colitis.—"Colitis with hemorrhage cured in two weeks. Bowel washed out with a 1% solution frequently and five drops of the pure oil three times a day taken internally."

re: Periostitis.—"Suppurating bruise of shin which appeared to be progressing to a condition of periostitis, checked in twenty-four hours using solution diluted 1—40 as a compress. Condition cured in one week by continuing this treatment."

re: Halitosis.—"In several cases of halitosis, especially after extraction, 5% or 1—20 dilution sprayed around the mouth gave almost instant relief within a few minutes."

re: Cuts, Bruises.—"For superficial cuts, bruises and small contusions, the oil is painted on 100% and left to dry. A scab forms and healing under the scab almost invariably takes place within a few days."

re: Vaginal Cleansing—"I find in the saponified form that it is a very pleasant and efficient preparation for using in douches and for cleaning up discharges from the cervix uteri."

re: Colds—"Personally free from colds during the year previously unknown. Personal friends relieved and cured of head and chest flu by inhaling (1) from a teaspoon of the pure oil in a pint of boiling water; (2) inserting a little of the pure oil in the nostril frequently."

re: Cleansing Wounds.—A senior surgeon in a Sydney hospital had the following observations: "The results obtained in a variety of conditions when it was first tried were most encouraging, a striking feature being that it dissolved pus and left the surface of infected wounds clean so that its germicidal action became more effective and without any apparent damage to the tissues....Dirty wounds, such as are frequently seen as the result of street accidents,....(the oil) will loosen and bring away the dirt which is usually ground in, and the tissues will remain fresh and retain their natural color."

Case Studies from Dr. David C. Evans, D.C.
of Evans Chiropractic in Littleton, Colorado

re: Athlete's Foot.—A 33-year old man, with a case of athlete's foot that left his feet raw, had been on prescribed medicine for three weeks with no noticeable improvement. Treatment prescribed: Dr. Evans instructed the man to use Tea Tree Oil three to four times a day. Results: Two days later feet almost healed completely. Followup: Due to his continuous work-outs in gyms, he uses oil or antiseptic cream as a preventative measure once a month.

re: Cuts and Burns.—A 32-year old male mechanic has cuts and burns continually. Treatment: Antiseptic Cream heals the burns, keeps the cuts clean and closed. Followup: Due to occupational cuts and burns, treatment with Tea Tree Oil and antiseptic cream continues on regular basis.

re: Acne.A 30-year-old female has minor cuts and facial blemishes possibly created by clogged pores. Treatment: Using Tea Tree Antiseptic Cream on cuts and face has helped clear up the skin.

re: Sunburn, Razorburn.—A 30-year-old male with razor burn and sunburn. Treatment: Tea Tree Antiseptic Cream has helped reduce the irritation and burn.

Dental Hygiene

Many Australian dentists use Tea Tree Oil as a mouthwash and for sterilizing cavities before filling. Studies have shown that washing the mouth out twice a day with a few drops of Tea Tree Oil will help to inhibit the growth of bacteria and reports state that gum bleeding has been greatly reduced and plaque controlled.

The Australian Journal of Dentistry reported that using Tea Tree Oil in dental hygiene and in surgery showed it to be an extremely effective antiseptic.

Toxicity Reports

Four cases of children swallowing twenty-five mls. of oil report no extreme side effects, except drowsiness and mild diarrhea. Symptoms disappeared within 24 hours.

Karen Cutter, naturopath in Sydney, took 120 drops of Tea Tree Oil daily for more than three months to demonstrate that her recommended dosages to patients associated with AIDS and systemic candida—sixty drops daily over six months time—produced no side-effects. **However, this type of treatment is not recommended unless under a physician's care.**

Personal Testimonials

"...my husband and I have been using the Tea Tree Oil for the past two years for a variety of ailments...came down with sore throats; we gargled with a few drops in water and within a few days the sore throat was gone...I got a severe sunburn...the Sun Soother lotion not only took away the pain but I never did blister or peel."

(T. L.—El Toro, California)

"After using Tea Tree Oil for the past two to three years in my busy herbalist/naturopathic practice...Tea Tree Oil works really well with...impetigo, the herpes simplex blisters, and most types of ulcerous tissue...it replaces anti-biotic powders. I carry your Tea Tree Oil in the car and in my bag where I use it as a 'First Aid Kit in a Bottle'."

(G. S.—herbal practitioner, Avalon, New South Wales)

≪ ≫

"...How grateful I am for your efforts and your book about Tea Tree Oil...I have very sensitive skin and am tired of many other medicines and products that seem to hurt and dull my senses. I have used Tea Tree Oil in taking sun, on my skin as a moisturizer...tonic on my hair...the oil helps soothe, heal and bring vitality to my skin, hair and my sense of life...I work in a very toxic profession, as an artist for almost twenty years...the oil helps alleviate the harm the leads, zincs and powerful solvents have on my system...looking forward to having the aid of this unique natural gift for the rest of my life..."

(C.G.—Montecito, California)

≪ ≫

"My husband contracted a severe cement dust allergy...he was confined to a wheelchair...(the) skin of his feet and calves was so tender...caused bleeding and great pain...our doctor advised that it was most likely that amputation of both legs below the knee would be necessary...I purchased a bottle and we rubbed it all over the affected area...Within two weeks the condition

had cleared up totally and...there has been no recurrence whatsoever...Your Tea Tree Oil is extraordinary."

(E. M.—Sydney, N.S.W.)

« »

"My clinic, 'The AIDS Alternative Health Project' is a donation-only clinic that serves 120 AIDS patients a week with 144 on a waiting list...Weekly visits to the clinic for treatment and a large homecare routine, much of which includes your Tea Tree Oil. Basically into every internal use—toothpaste, drops on tongue, in vaporizer, enemas, suppositories...While not a cure, I feel absolute success in candida control, skin infections, etc."

(A. S.—Ac.T., Chicago, IL)

« »

"Just a quick note to tell you how great your Tea Tree Oil has helped my skin problem clear up."

(T. A.—San Marcus, California)

« »

"My son, Rudie, went to summer camp and came home just eaten up with mosquito bites all over his body. He was scratching them making matters worse. I applied your Tea Tree Oil and in just 20 minutes the itching stopped and the next morning all was well."

(C. C.—Dallas, Texas)

« »

"Thank you, thank you, for the marvelous Tea Tree Oil. I have been suffering from cold sores for years and they get quite bad at times to the point of leaving scar tissue

27

on my face. My last bout with this problem was much better, thanks to your Tea Tree Oil. In fact, as I felt it coming on, I started using the Tea Tree Oil and it never developed into a sore."

(C. D.—Rockwall, Texas)

≪ ≫

"While at a health food trade show in Las Vegas three years ago, I learned about the amazing healing applications of Tea Tree Oil. One area that particularly interested me was dental applications. At the age of sixty-five, I was suffering from receding and bleeding gums. I purchased some oil and decided to put it to the test.

I took the Tea Tree Oil to my dentist and had a full checkup. I told him that I was going to rinse my mouth out twice a day with three drops of Tea Tree Oil in a small cup of water, for three to five minutes.

I must tell you that my dentist would get blood at almost every place on my gums. I also gave up flossing. The plan was to have a checkup every thirty days for a prolonged period of time. My first checkup after thirty days already began to show improvement. My dentist could draw blood in only six spots. In sixty days, there was no bleeding at all, even with the gums being deeply gouged. After thirteen months of treatment, the gums stopped bleeding and the receding gums had returned to normal. The dentist said that the plaque and calculus had been reduced 75-80%. Tea Tree Oil saved my teeth. Aloha!"

(B.Mc.—Oahu, Hawaii)

"Thank you from the bottom, top and sides of my heart! Your Tea Tree Oil is...wonderful...As a person with AIDS, I take massive doses of different drugs. These drugs dry my skin. The Tea Tree Oil/Cream helps to reverse this dryness and makes life a whole lot better..."

(J.I.—Washington, D.C.)

◄ ►

"I consider our discovery of...Tea Tree Oil...to be one of the better things that happened to us in 1990. I've had arthritis for several years and find I get the greatest relief by applying Tea Tree to the affected joint (or area.) A gargle solution of two or three drops of Tea Tree Oil in a 1/4 cup of water certainly nips a threatening sore throat in the bud.

I have always had a problem with plaque buildup on my teeth and have them cleaned every six months for that. After three months of adding a couple of drops of the oil to the toothpaste before brushing, I've experienced no plaque buildup and my teeth are definitely whiter.

Cuts, burns, abrasions and insect bites heal so much more quickly with Tea Tree Oil. I use the antiseptic lotion for vaginal cleanliness, as well as for extremely dry skin. My husband particularly likes Tea Tree soap and toothpaste."

(F.B.—Carlsbad, California)

◄ ►

"Thanks for the information on Tea Tree Oil. I am passing along the pertinent data to my vet...I am sure she will be interested, especially after seeing what it is doing with the viral growth on my horse's back. This is

29

a viral growth called a sarcoid and it appears also to be diminishing with the use of the Tea Tree Oil. The other bump which I eliminated doesn't have a name that I know of, but is like an infected ingrown hair. We continue to make these disappear on both of our horses' backs with Tea Tree Oil..."

(J.E.—Scottsdale, Arizona)

≪ ≫

"To prevent dehydration of the skin in the airplane I use Tea Tree Antiseptic Lotion—I don't know what I would do without it."

(B. D.—Airline Captain of 29 years)

≪ ≫

"About four years ago we began to experience infestations of 'kissing bugs' or cone-nosed beetles in our house during May and June. The bugs always seemed to bite me at night while I was asleep. The next morning, I would have a huge lump at the location of the bite, and it would be itchy and painful. It generally took 2-3 days for the lump to go away. Nothing of the medications I used seemed to help, until I tried Tea Tree Oil. When I first discovered a bite, I rubbed in some of the oil and kept doing so at frequent intervals. Relief of the itching was almost immediate, and within 6-8 hours of the first application of the oil, the swelling was drastically reduced. I definitely plan to keep my medicine cabinet stocked with Tea Tree Oil."

(D.B.—Fountain Hills, Arizona)

≪ ≫

Images

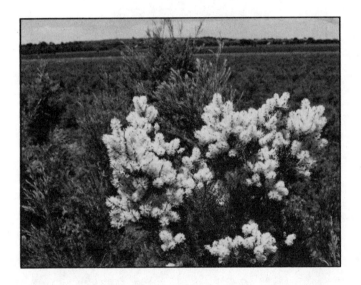

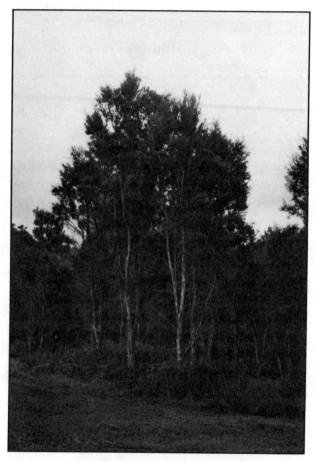

THE HEALING TREES
A natural stand of Tea Trees in the bush country
of New South Wales, Australia.

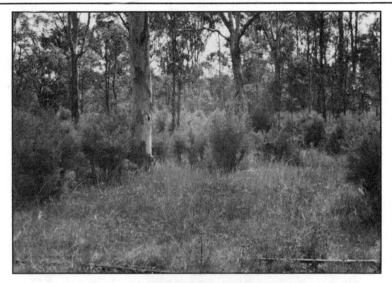

NEW GROWTH
Tea Tree Plantation showing seedlings among mature trees:
Clarence and Richmond River region.

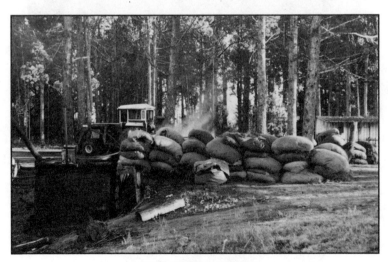

NEW HARVEST
Freshly gathered Tea Tree leaves are delivered to the still
site to be processed, wrapped in Hessian sacks.

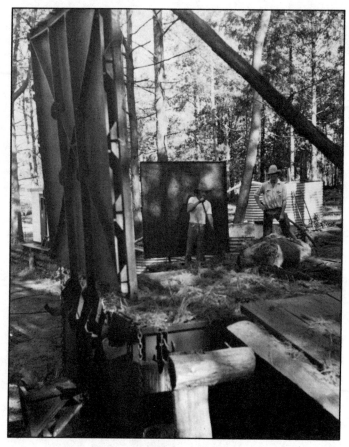

PROCESSING
Cut Tea Tree leaves about to be distilled.

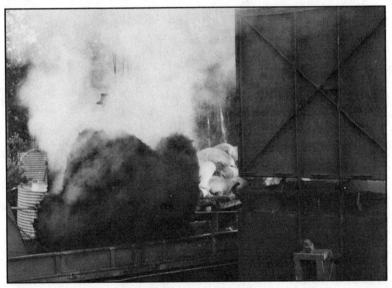

DISTILLING
The distilling process takes some hours to complete, the
essential oil being obtained from the leaves through steaming.

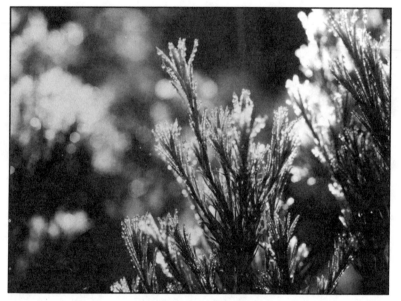

NATURE'S GIFT
Sunlight glistens off oil gathered on the delicate leaves of a
Tea Tree.

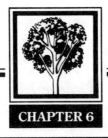

CHAPTER 6

Beauty, Face and Body Care

Face and Body Care

Many French cosmetic manufacturers, and recently U.S. companies, are using the Tea Tree essential oil in toiletry and cosmetic formulations. Tea Tree's spicy aroma adds appeal when mixed into soaps, shampoos, lotions and perfumes. Tea Tree Oil contains antiseptic and antifungal properties. Thus skin creams that contain as little as 2% Tea Tree Oil will help to combat bacteria. Skin also takes on a youthful glow. The oil's penetration helps to oxygenate skin cells while aiding in the repair of damaged skin caused by sun, acne, dry skin, fungus and various other skin ailments. In fact, the U.S. government has approved the use of Tea Tree Oil in cosmetic formulations. The oil contains very low levels of toxicity. Tea Tree Oil is non-irritating to all areas of the body and at times, depending on the application and treatment, will slough off dead tissue to allow healthy skin to appear.

In this day and age, more people are becoming susceptible to viral conditions such as cold sores. Since cold sores usually appear on the face and around the mouth, the infected individual may become self-conscious about the outbreak. Normally, cold sores can be controlled by applying a few drops of pure Tea Tree Oil onto the infected area at the onset. The oil will help to keep the cold sore from manifesting.

Dermatitis, dry skin, fungus, corns, and athlete's foot are just a few skin problems that we all face at one time or another. Generally, dry skin brushing and using a body lotion with Tea

Tree Oil added will help to repair and smooth the injured skin. Bathing in Tea Tree Oil is soothing for tired muscles. Adding ten drops of the oil to a warm tub and soaking for twenty minutes will be very therapeutic and soothing. It is not necessary to use a lot of oil. I once had a call from a woman who added an entire ounce to her tub, sat in hot water for one hour and her skin turned bright red. Remember, a little goes a long way.

After shaving or waxing, apply several drops of the oil on the newly waxed or shaved area. It helps to cut down on redness or swelling. A lotion with a few drops of Tea Tree Oil in it will also work well. Ingrown hairs can be eliminated by massaging the oil into the skin. This method is effective for both men and women.

Hair Care

Both women and men tease, color, mousse, blow-dry and perm their hair. Not only is the hair left in dry condition, but the hair follicle itself can be blocked, creating further problems which often create hair thinning and loss. A Tea Tree Oil shampoo with a 2% amount of Tea Tree Oil (ten drops to a eight-ounce bottle) will help to unblock clogged hair follicles, moisturize the hair and keep the scalp free of bacteria and fungal problems. As far back as 1939, Tea Tree Oil has been used as a dandruff treatment. There have also been reports that by massaging the oil into the scalp, new hair growth was promoted.

Hair Treatments for Children

When both of my grandchildren were little, my daughter called and asked if she could use the Tea Tree Oil as a treatment for cradle cap. I suggested that she take one part of pure oil and mix it with ten parts of another oil, such as almond oil. She could gently massage the oil into the baby's scalp and leave it on for a few minutes. She could then follow up with the Tea Tree shampoo wash. My daughter called me back a few days later and reported that the cradle cap was gone!

It seems that at the beginning of every school year, there is an outbreak of head lice among school children. Since headlice is contagious, it can be widespread. I spoke once to a Dallas school nurse who voiced concern regarding the use of chemically-based shampoos that was the standard treatment for children's head lice. She expressed a great deal of interest in being able to offer the Tea Tree Oil as a natural substitute. The following treatment for removal of head lice is recommended. Apply five to ten drops of the pure oil to a shampoo and massage this mixture thoroughly into the child's scalp every day until the eggs are removed. Also, in between shampoos, a few drops of the oil can be massaged into the scalp. Do not rinse out. Brushes, combs, bedding and towels can be soaked in a Tea Tree Oil solution to help sterilize and prevent further lice manifestation. Normally, 1/4 oz. of oil added to a tub of water should do the trick.

Nail Care

Within the last ten years, Deborah's Nail Care Center in Texas has observed an increase in the occurrence of paronychia, a fungal infection which appears on fingernails and toenails. She feels this is due to the popularity of acrylic and silk nail applications. Many women have their nails redone every two weeks; sometimes when the nails are applied, moisture may get trapped in the nail bed. If this happens, a lifting of the nail bed may occur within a week and a half. If left untreated, a fungus could develop. Deborah has witnessed three stages of nail fungus:

Stage 1: If moisture occurs and the nail begins to lift and is left untreated, a light green stain will appear on the nail bed if ignored.

Stage 2: The nail bed will turn dark green.
Stage 3: The nail bed will eventually turn black. A light yellow tinge usually indicates a nail fungus as well.

There have been horror stories told of women refusing to treat their nail fungus and asking their nail salon to cut back the infected nail and slap another nail on top. Many salons may refuse to do this due to the poor condition of the nail. Deborah's salon has witnessed dramatic results applying Tea Tree Oil on, around and under the nail bed, rubbing in several drops twice a day. For cases of mildew, she uses a mixture of a few drops of Tea Tree Oil in liquid soap. This is massaged onto the nail plate and then all residue washed off. It is important to have nails free of any oil residue so that the new nail application will adhere properly. To remove nail stains, buff the infected nail with iodine and Tea Tree Oil. The nail will dry to a milky white color. Buff off the milky white to remove all the stain from the nail.

Aromatherapy

What are essential oils? Essential oils are the essences of plant material which are extracted by a steam distillation process. Essential oils can be mixed with vegetable oils or alcohol. They are blended into perfumes, bath oils and cosmetics to name a few. The oils help to balance, rejuvenate and stimulate the body and skin. Essential oils can be applied into massage lotions, bath oils, diffusers, facial masks, saunas, compresses, and perfumes. Each oil contains its own essential quality. The French gathered clinical data on the oil in the mid-1980's. (Refer to Clinical Data chapter.)

Robert Tisserand, an English Aromatherapist, has discussed Tea Tree Oil in his books, *Aromatherapy for Everyone* and *The Art of Aromatherapy.* In the *International Journal of Aromatherapy,* February 1988, Mr. Tisserand called Tea Tree Oil one of the most exciting essential oils to emerge.

Tea Tree Oil in Aromatherapy

Tea Tree Oil has been recognized as a powerful antiseptic and fungicide and shown to be twelve times stronger than carbolic acid, the world's number one antiseptic. Arthur Penfold, the English chemist who discovered and did laboratory studies on the Melaleuca alternifolia in 1923, confirmed that Tea Tree Oil was indeed much stronger than carbolic acid. Thus, Tea Tree is excellent as a **first aid oil** to help alleviate fungus on finger and toenails and on the skin. **As a massage** it can be blended with other oils to give the skin a refreshing feeling and to help keep the skin clean and healthy. **As a bath soak,** ten drops in a tub will help to alleviate sore and injured muscles and joints as well as infections of the skin. I have applied several drops in the **humidifier** to keep the air in my home clean. I have a **diffuser** I purchased several years ago from an essential oil company. By putting a few drops of the Tea Tree Oil into the diffuser, the aroma must be likened to sitting in a grove of Tea Trees in the Australian bush. My daughter has used a few drops in the **vaporizer** which gives tremendous relief to the children when they come down with the sniffles.

Tea Tree Oil definitely can be added to the list of other fine essential oils as a great contribution to aromatherapy. Please remember to store the pure oil in amber glass bottles to protect from heat and light, and keep in a cool area of your home. If you mix the Tea Tree Oil into other lotions, plastic is suitable to use. **Refer to the First Aid usage chapter for more Tea Tree Oil applications.**

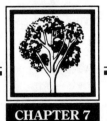

CHAPTER 7

Animal Care

Horse Care

I n the spring of 1991, I received a call from a woman named Juanita Engoji. Juanita was calling to ask if I could supply some Tea Tree Oil to be used on her thoroughbred horse, Marshall, for a virus condition known as a sarcoid.

Because the sarcoid was located on Marshall's back, every time he was ridden, the rubbing of the saddle and pad caused irritation and bleeding.

About six weeks after I sent her the oil, Juanita asked if I could come to her ranch so that she could show me how effective the Tea Tree Oil had been in treating the virus. When I arrived, her horse was in the final stages of treatment. Observing the sarcoid, I noticed flaking and a little bit of whiteness, which indicated that the Tea Tree Oil was sloughing off the dead tissue and drying up the virus. There was no infection to be seen.

Juanita told me that she has been using several drops of Tea Tree Oil 2—3 times a day, rubbing it right onto the raised area. It did not seem to bother Marshall to have it applied in such a manner.

In the initial stages, a sarcoid appears as a black bump on the horse. It is normally raised, perhaps 1/2" high depending on the extent of the virus. If left untreated, the sarcoid will spread so it is very important to be able to treat it as soon as possible.

Traditional treatments for sarcoids would be injections with the actual virus into the horse. However, Juanita's veterinarian said that the virus normally comes back. Juanita is very interested to find out if the Tea Tree Oil treatment will prevent the sarcoid from coming back. If it starts reappearing, she can apply the Tea Tree Oil immediately to stop it from growing any larger.

Juanita also experienced an incident with Marshall bruising his right front hoof to the point where he couldn't apply any pressure on it. Juanita's vet suggested an epsom salt soak for the hoof. Juanita added several drops of the Tea Tree Oil along with the epsom salts in a bucket of water and for a few minutes twice a day soaked Marshall's foot. Within three days she noticed immediate relief where he could apply pressure on his foot once again. The inflammation and bruising were greatly reduced.

A similar treatment uses a boot called an Easyboot. Cotton soaked with epsom salts and Tea Tree Oil is put around the hoof. The Easyboot is then clamped over the hoof and left for one to two days. At that time, a freshly saturated cotton pad is applied and the Easyboot replaced. This method reduces inflammation and any abscess and within three to four days, the treatment can be discontinued.

Juanita and her husband told me they also use Tea Tree Oil for ingrown hairs on their horses' backs. I asked them what would create ingrown hairs on a horse and their explanation was that if the saddle pad is placed on the horse against the grain of the hair, it creates an abrasion which may cause ingrown hairs. Rubbing several drops of the Tea Tree Oil into the ingrown hairs will keep infection from occurring and allows the ingrown hairs to work their way out. Also, proper grooming and making sure the saddle pads are laid with the grain of the horse's hair will help.

Recently, I visited an Arabian horse farm in Scottsdale, Arizona to talk the groomers and the trainers regarding a fungus that has been appearing on some of the horses. Apparently the reason that horses, especially in Arizona, get fungus is because they are in their stalls for 22—23 hours a day and the other couple of hours they are put on hot walkers and exercised. The groomers have had success using Tea Tree Oil to eliminate the fungus. I looked at a horse that had developed a fungus on the inside hind leg; by the time I saw it, the area was already flaking and clearing up.

Horse owners have also found a use for Tea Tree Oil as a fly repellent. In the summer when the heat climbs up to over 100 degrees in Arizona, the flies—especially the horse flies—come out in numbers and they will bother the horses tremendously. Application of Tea Tree Oil full strength around the horse's eyes, face and body helps to repel flies. The oil also acts as a preventative measure against infections or irritations of the skin due to the fly bites.

A letter received from Mrs. Karen Leucht of Stapylton, Queensland dated February 5, 1988 emphasizes the value of Tea Tree Oil in treating more serious wounds:

"On New Year's Eve, a mare of mine had an operation on her shoulder requiring stitching. Within a week, the stitching had busted open and the wound was infected with staph. The wound was deep, through the flesh and muscle and about the size of a bread and butter plate. The vet gave the mare very little chance of surviving and they couldn't stitch the wound and he said the staph infection would spread to her blood system. I started to spray Tea Tree Oil directly on the wound and within 14 days, the mare was left with only a 1-2 inch scar completely healed. The proud flesh was not burnt by the oil and I cannot believe its healing properties. My vet and other local vets are amazed and said they want copies of my photos as well so they can begin recommending it to customers."

Dog and Cat Care

While living in Santa Barbara, California, I discovered that dogs and cats suffer immeasurably from allergies that create the

"Santa Barbara itch." I witnessed my 14-year-old cat, Pepper, practically going crazy by itching constantly. Out came the Tea Tree Oil. I would smooth a few drops, diluted with water, onto her skin. I could practically hear her "meow" a sigh of relief.

Tea Tree Oil is an excellent flea repellent. You won't eliminate all the pesky critters; however, by spraying the carpet with a Tea Tree Oil mixture, it will help to control the fleas. It is a good idea to take the pets outside before you wash them with the Tea Tree shampoo so the fleas can jump off there rather than in the house. This goes for brushing their coats with the Tea Tree Oil as well. Bathing your pet once a week helps to curb skin irritations.

Four years ago, I received a call from a friend named Mark Blumenthal. Mark has been associated with the health food industry for a very long time and also writes a publication called *Herbalgram* and contributes many articles to the health food magazines in the United States. He had asked if I could give him some oil so that he could use it on a cat that had appeared at his door one day wearing a flea collar that had gotten caught up under her right leg. The collar had rubbed the skin raw and created a large opening. Mark removed the collar and doused the area with a generous amount of the Tea Tree Oil. He used the oil for about two weeks and also used a comfrey lanolin ointment. Mark said that the wound healed and that there was no scar.

Recently, a cat clinic called to share the following interesting event:
Several cats had developed ringworm; the symptoms included loss of hair, depression and nausea. The medicine normally prescribed would eat away their bone marrow. The cats would have to be shaved, given a sulphur bath and have their blood tested. Talk about trauma! So the clinic made a formula of Tea Tree Oil with olive oil. Black walnut and cateput oil were also

used in the treatment. The cats responded well and an immediate improvement was noted.

From my experience with cats, I would recommend using a very small amount of Tea Tree Oil or diluting it with water or a cold-pressed oil such as almond oil. Cats seem to be more sensitive than dogs to certain skin treatments.

Case Studies

In the spring of 1988, the Veterinary Superintendent of St. Ives Veterinary Clinic submitted an animal testing report to Thursday Plantation, a leading manufacturer of Australian Tea Tree products.

For the previous sixteen to eighteen months, treatment trials were prescribed using a Tea Tree Oil shampoo supplied by Thursday Plantation. There was a variety of skin ailments, most noticeably of an allergic and/or pruritic nature.

Annabelle Olsson, the Superintendent, reported that the Tea Tree Oil shampoo was a success as an "anti-itch" treatment and that in 80% of the cases, pruritus was controlled or diminished. She also noted that regular bathing with the shampoo helped decrease the flea population, as well as improve the condition of the animals' coats.

The following case histories summarize the animal testing that was reported by Annabelle Olsson:

Case No. 1: Labrador retriever, 6 years of age, spayed female.
History—Eczema and fleas.
Therapy—Tea Tree Oil shampoo once a week. Within two weeks, coat condition improved. Flea rinse only required now every two weeks.

Case No. 2: Cat, 10-year old neutered male.
History—Chronic dermatitis and "hot spots" behind ears.
Therapy—Tea Tree Oil shampoo every 1-2 weeks. Also, pure

Tea Tree Oil directly on the coat. The dermatitis was reduced dramatically.

Case No. 3: Australian cattle dog, 4 years old, spayed female.

History—Flea allergy and trauma.

Therapy—Tea Tree Oil shampoo weekly. For the last six months, fleas are minimal.

Case No. 4: Pekingese, 14-year-old male.

History—Fungal lesions on neck and chest.

Therapy—Tea Tree Oil shampoo daily. Tea Tree Oil applied after bath. Within five days, improvement dramatic. In three weeks, lesions completely gone.

Case No. 5: Cocker Spaniel/Poodle. 8-year-old male.

History—Chronic flea allergy dermatitis. Animal attacking its tail.

Therapy—Iodine scrub, Tea Tree Oil shampoo weekly. Reduced problem within two weeks.

Case No. 6: Golden retriever, 9-year-old spayed female.

History—Nervous dog with skin allergies. Fleas severe in summer.

Therapy—Tea Tree Oil shampoo twice a week. Owner discontinued treatment against veterinarian's advice.

Case No. 7: Labrador/Setter, 8-year-old male.

History—Chronic pruritus and hair loss on rump, flanks, thighs and abdomen.

Therapy—Tea Tree Oil shampoo weekly. Within three weeks, hair began to regrow. Six months later, dog has healthy coat and receives regular Tea Tree Oil shampoos.

Case No. 8: Cat, 14-year old neutered male.

History—Flea allergy dermatitis.

Therapy—Tea Tree Oil shampoo 1-2 times a week. Hair began to regrow within two weeks.

It must be noted that in all eight cases, the animals had been treated with drugs such as megoestrol or prednisolone during their previous treatments. In some cases, steroids were continued for only a short period of time. Preventative maintenance including healthy diets and clean environment were important steps in the animals' recoveries as well.

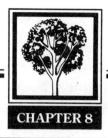

CHAPTER 8

Products With Tea Tree Oil

S oaps—Tea Tree Oil soap has shown to be very effective for skin blemishes, irritations, and as a general antiseptic. Many people with sensitive skin have reported the soap to be effective as well as mild, not causing skin irritation. Using the soap on a daily basis would be beneficial for acne, cuts, abrasions, foot conditions, fungal irritations, and rashes.

Shampoo—A Tea Tree shampoo helps to control dandruff, itchy scalp, ringworm, lice, and seborrhea (see Chapter 6). Using shampoo either on a daily basis or alternating with other naturally based shampoos is recommended.

Antiseptic Cream—A therapeutic cream containing at least 5% Tea Tree Oil helps heal nappy rash, sunburns, cuts, mosquito bites, rashes, Athlete's Foot, and a number of other skin irritations.

Douche—Yeast infections and candida have become prevalent in today's society because of eating habits, stress, accumulation of antibiotic treatments, moist conditions, etc. (See Chapter 3, the text by Dr. Paul Belaiche of France in 1985.) A pessary product can be used vaginally and in the anal passage for difficulties such as hemorrhoids. A 2% solution of Tea Tree Oil in a cocoa butter base has been effective in inhibiting the growth of infection without disturbing the body's natural flora. Recommended use should be under medical supervision. A Tea Tree Oil douche has also been used for infections. Eight to ten drops of oil in a pint of purified or distilled water and douching in between pessary applications seems to help in reducing irritation, discomfort, and infection.

Tea Tree Toothpaste—Tea Tree toothpaste may prove to be effective for gingivitis, halitosis, plaque control and pyorrhea, as well as in dental surgery (refer to Case Studies, Chapter 5.) Many Australian dentists use Tea Tree Oil as a mouthwash and to sterilize cavities before filling. Studies have shown that washing the mouth out twice a day with a few drops of Tea Tree Oil will help to inhibit the growth of bacteria and reports state that gum bleeding has been greatly reduced and plaque controlled. Thus Tea Tree Oil dental products would appear to be of great benefit.

Tea Tree Oil Deodorant—Many of the deodorant products out today contain aluminum and other ingredients that may or may not be beneficial. Here again is another area where Tea Tree Oil can play a role as a healthier alternative. Because Tea Tree Oil is 10-13 times stronger than carbolic acid (once considered the Number One antiseptic in the world) a Tea Tree Oil deodorant may help to minimize risk of bacteria build-up and heal razor burns as well.

Anti-Itch Pet Shampoos—Skin allergies in animals lead to itching and chaffing of the skin. Many animals have scratched themselves raw. A pet shampoo, if used once or twice a week, will help heal the irritations, stop the itching, and promote a healthy coat. Use of several drops of Tea Tree Oil directly on the infected area will help clear the problem. This can be done daily. Ticks have backed out of animals' skin when anointed with the oil. Fleas can be controlled as well. Be sure to leave the pet shampoo on for three to five minutes before you rinse. This product is beneficial for dogs, cats and horses. This is an excellent alternative to the toxic "dips" done in many veterinary offices.

Tea Tree Marketplace—Several Australian and American companies are now producing an entire line of Tea Tree products and are adding the oil to their existing or new formulations. Sun screens, mouthwash, lozenges, massage oils, creams and lotions are now appearing on the health food shelves throughout the

United States. One company boasts the production of over sixty products made with Tea Tree Oil which include biodegradable household cleaning items.

Tea Tree Oil is also being used by chiropractors for the relief of muscle tightness as well as for skin irritations. Another Tea Tree product that proves useful for professionals as well as for individuals is a salve for sore muscles. Tea Tree Oil products have been used in Australia by naturopaths for some time now for the treatment of thrush. Switzerland uses the oil to control infections in hospitals; an Australian industrial company uses it in a product to help sterilize air-conditioning and venting systems in public buildings to aid in the control of Legionnaire's Disease.

Meanwhile Tea Tree Oil is becoming visible in the mass marketplace. Hair salon products include a Tea Tree Shampoo. Mail order catalogues are beginning to include Tea Tree Oil and products in their lines. With the increased awareness of herbal products in mainstream consciousness, the immediate future holds exciting possibilities for Tea Tree Oil in many different marketplaces.

Safety Data

Identification

Product Name: Oil of Melaleuca alternifolia
Synonyms: Tea Tree Oil
Chemical Composition: Essential oil containing terpinene-4-ol, other terpene alcohols, sesquiterpines, 1, 8 cineole, p-cymene, etc.
CAS No.: 68647-73-4

Physical and Chemical Composition Data

Physical State: Liquid
Color: Colorless to Pale Yellow
Odor: Myristic
Specific Gravity: 20/20°C: 0.890 to 0.906
Refractive Index @ 20°C: 1.475 to 1.482
Solubility: Insoluble in Water/Soluble in Alcohol
Boiling Point: Not Determined
Vapor Density: (Air=1) > 1
Saponification Value: 2-3
1,8 Cineole Content: Shall not exceed 10%
Terpinen-4-ol Content: Shall be at least 36%

Fire and Explosion Hazard Data

Flash Point (Open Cup): 140°C
Extinguishing Media: Dry Chemical Foam
Special Fire Fighting
   Procedures: None Known
Unusual Fire & Explosion
Hazards None Known

Reactivity Data

Stability: Presents no significant reactivity hazard. Stable even at elevated temperatures and pressures.

Incompatibility: Solvent—avoid contact with plastics, oil based paints, ink etc., or storage in plastic containers.

Hazardous Polymerization: Does not occur

Toxicity and Health Hazard Data

Toxicity: No cases of Acute or Chronic Toxicity reported.

Health Hazards: None Known

First Aid: Eye contact—irrigate with water.
Skin contact—wash with mild soap and water.
Ingestion—drink copious quantities of water.

Personal Protection Information

Respiratory: None required

Ventilation: Good room ventilation, local exhaust optional

Protective Glove: Oil resistant gloves optional

Eye Protection: Safety glasses optional

Other Protective Equipment: None required

Special Storage and Handling Precaution

Store in Stainless Steel or Glass Containers ONLY
Bottle should be well capped and kept in cool place.

Glossary, Part A

Tea Tree Oil and Tea Tree related products are effective on the following conditions. Apply sparingly, directly to the site of the problem. Dilute if desirable.

Arthritis—Inflammation of one or more joints. Swelling, redness of the skin, and impaired motion. Two types: 1) osteo; chronic disease involving joints, especially weight-bearing joints; 2) rheumatoid; chronic systemic disease characterized by inflammatory changes in joints that may result in crippling.

Boil (Furuncle)—A localized swelling and inflammation of the skin resulting from the infection of a sebaceous gland.

Candida Albicans—Formerly called monilia albicans. Yeast-like fungus that resides in vagina, alimentary tract. A small oval budding fungus. May result in candidiasis occurring in moist areas of the body, mouth, lungs, vagina, skin, nails, or intestines.

Carbuncles—A collection of boils with multiple draining channels. Caused by staphylococcus aureaus. Usually terminates in extensive sloughing of the skin. Characterized by a painful node, covered by tight red skin that later becomes thin and discharges pus. Commonly found on nape of neck, upper back, or buttocks.

Cold Sore (Herpes Simplex)—A viral infection causing inflammation of the skin, usually on mouth or lips, and characterized by collections of small blisters.

Corn (clavus)—Area of hard thickened skin on or between toes. May form an inverted pyramid pressing into deeper skin layers, causing pain.

Cradle Cap—Dermatitis of a newborn, usually appearing on scalp, face, and head. Thick, yellowish crusted lesions will develop on the scalp and scaling will appear behind ears.

Dermatitis—An inflammation of the skin caused by an outside agent. The skin is red and itchy, and small blisters may develop. Causes may include soaps or detergents, sunlight, allergies, or hot weather. In about 70% of the cases, a family history exists.

Gingivitis—Inflammation of the gums, redness, swelling, and bleeding.

Hemorrhoids (Piles)—Enlarged varicose veins in the wall of the anus, due to constipation or diarrhea.

Nasal Ulcer—An open sore or lesion of the mucous membrane accompanied by sloughing of inflamed tissue.

Plantar Wart (Verruca Plantaris)—Wart occurring in skin on sole of the foot, usually at base of the toes. Caused by a virus. Because of pressure, these warts are painful.

Poison Ivy—Dermatitis resulting from irritation or sensitization of the skin by the resin of the poison ivy plant. Reaction to poison ivy contact may appear several hours or several days afterwards. Moderate itching or burning sensation followed by small blisters. Blisters will usually burst and be followed by oozing and crusting.

Poison Oak—A climbing vine, related to poison ivy.

Psoriasis—A chronic skin disease with itchy, scaly red patches forming on elbows, forearms, knees, legs, scalp, and other parts of the body. Affects 1-2% of the population.

Rash—An eruption on the skin characterized by redness and welts with very little elevation.

Scabies (sarcoptes scabiei)—Skin infection caused by the itch mite. Severe itching (especially at night), red papules, and secondary infection. Female mite tunnels into the skin to lay eggs. Newly hatched eggs are passed from person to person. Common areas affected are the groin, penis, nipples, and skin between fingers. Clothing and bedding should be dis-infested.

Shingles (Herpes Zoster)—Viral infection of the nervous system characterized by pain and blisters. Blistering usually subsides within a three-week period. The virus also causes chickenpox in children.

Sinusitis—Inflammation of one or more of the mucus-lined, air spaces. It is often caused by infection spreading from the nose. Symptoms may include headache and tenderness.

Tick—A blood-sucking parasite belonging to the order of arthropods that includes mites. Tick bites can cause skin lesions.

Tropical Ulcer (Naga Sore)—An indolent (inactive, painless) ulcer of lower extremities (feet or legs) usually occurring in hot, humid climates. May be due to bacteria, nutrition, or environment. A large, open sloughing sore usually develops.

Wart (Verruca)—A small (often hard) benign growth caused by a virus. Occurring on hands, fingers, face, elbows, and knees.

If condition persists following prescribed treatment, discontinue and consult a physician.

Glossary, Part B

Tea Tree Oil—Melaleucae alternifolia

Composition. Naturally occurring essential oil, colorless to pale yellow, distilled from leaves of Melaleuca alternifolia, consisting chiefly of terpinenes, cymones, pinenes, terpineols, cineol, sesquinterpenes, and sequiterpene alcohols. Pleasant characteristic odor with a terebinthinate taste.

Action. Pure Tea Tree Oil conforming to Australian standard A.S.D 175, revised 1985, is a powerful broad-range antiseptic, fungicide, and bactericide. (In fact, Tea Tree Oil is four to five times stronger than household antiseptics.) Its bacterial action is increased in the presence of blood, serum, pus, and necrotic tissue. It is able to penetrate deeply into infected tissue and pus, mix with these, and cause them to slough off while leaving a healthy surface. The oil has a very low toxicity, and is virtually a non-irritant even to sensitive tissues. Because of its lower cineole level, Tea Tree Oil is less toxic and less irritating than eucalyptus oil.

Indications. Cuts, scratches, abrasions, burns, sunburn, prickly heat, insect bites, scalds, allergic and itching dermatoses, napkin and cosmetic rashes, senile, anal and genital pruritus, and lesions caused by herpes simplex virus including herpes labialis and herpes progenitalis. Impetigo contagiosa, furunculosis, psoriasis, and infected seborrhoeic dermatitis. Ringworm of scalp (microsporum canis), tropical ringworm (triphyton), becubitis and stasis ulcers, paronychia, oral thrush (candidiasis),

57

tinea pedis, bromidrosis, and infestation with head, body, or pubic lice. As a gargle, throat spray, and nasal spray. Treatment of cutaneous staphylococcal reservoirs, boils and pimples. Pyorrhea, gingivitis, halitosis, and bronchial and sinus congestion. Gynecological conditions such as trichomonal vaginitis, moniliasis, and endocervicitis.

Precautions. *Pure oil will dissolve certain plastics. Store in glass containers only in a cool place.* Extremely sensitive skin may need dilutions of the pure oil. Dilutions of 1:250 are still bacteriostatic against pathogenic streptococci and staphylococci, typhous, pneumococcus, and gonococcus.

Clinical Data

February 29, 1988
Re: Disinfectant test: T.G.A. (Otion D) Antiseptic Grade

A sample marked as detailed below was received on the 8/2/1988 and was analysed as directed with the following results:

Sample: Tea Tree Oil, 80% Dispersible
EML S/N: 88/110.2

Test	Count (Orgs/ml)	Growth in Recovery Broth	Results
A. Pseudomonas aeruginosa NCTC 6749			
Day 1	2.6×10^6	- - - - -	PASS
Day 2	6.0×10^6	+ + - - -	PASS
Day 3	6.7×10^6	+ - - - -	PASS
B. Proteus vulgaris NCTC 4635			
Day 1	2.9×10^6	- - - - -	PASS
Day 2	8.7×10^6	- - - - -	PASS
Day 3	4.1×10^6	- - - - -	PASS
C. Escherischia coli NCTC 8196			
Day 1	6.0×10^6	- - - - -	PASS
Day 2	6.1×10^6	- - - - -	PASS
Day 3	6.5×10^6	- - - - -	PASS
D. Staphylococcus aureus NCTC 4163			
Day 1	5.4×10^6	+ + - - -	PASS
Day 2	6.2×10^6	- - - - -	PASS
Day 3	5.9×10^6	- - - - -	PASS

The product marked 'Tea Tree Oil, 80% Dispersible' was found to PASS the T.G.A. test Option D at a NEAT dilution.

20th August 1987
Re: MIC determination of Tea Tree Oil against Fungi.

Sample description: 100% Pure Tea Tree Oil Batch "0166"

Results

TEST ORGANISM	CONCENTRATION OF SAMPLE IN TEST DILUENT (% v/v)						
	0.0	0.25	0.50	0.75	1.00	1.25	1.50
Aspergillus niger	+	+	+	-	-	-	
Candida albicans	+	+	-	-	-	-	
Trichophyton mentagrophytes	+	+	+	-	-	-	

Notes: Aspergillus niger ATCC 16404
   Candida albicans ATCC 10231
   Trichophyton mentagrophytes var. interdigitale

Method The agar dilution method was used. Using T.S.A. agar containing the sample at the concentrations detailed above. These plates were then streaked with the appropriate organisms. The plates were incubated at 30°C for 5 days and then examined for growth.

August 20, 1987
Re: MIC determination of Tea Tree Oil against Legionella spp.
Sample description: 100% Pure Tea Tree Oil Batch "0166"

RESULTS

TEST ORGANISM	CONCENTRATION OF SAMPLE IN TEST DILUENT (% v/v)						
	0.0	0.25	0.50	0.75	1.00	1.25	1.50
L. pneumophilia Gp. 1	+	+	+	+			
L. pneumophilia Gp. 2	+	+	+	-	-	-	-
L. pneumophilia Gp. 4	+	+	+	+	-	-	-
L. dumoffii	+	+	+	-	-	-	-
L. germanii	+	+		+			

Notes All above are Legionella species.

Method

The agar dilution method was used. Using alpha DCYE media (Oxoid) containing the sample at the concentrations detailed above. These plates were then streaked with the appropriate organisms. The plates were incubated in 6% CO_2 at 35°C for 28 days, and were examined at 7 day intervals.

TEA TREE OIL

19th January 1987
Re: Microbiological Testing

Dear Sir,

A sample marked "Tea Tree Oil Batch 0166" was received in December, and analysed as directed according to the T.G.A. test for hospital grade dirty conditions (OptB).

The tests were performed in triplicate, utilising fresh cultures and solutions on each occasion. The results were found to be as follows:

Sample: Tea Tree Oil 0166   Dilution   NEAT

Test	Count (orgs/ml)	Growth in Recovery broths		RESULT
Pseudomonas aeruginosa NCTC 6749				
Day 1	1.9×10^9	- - - + -	- - - + +	PASS
Day 2	6.5×10^8	- - - - -	- - - - -	PASS
Day 3	8.2×10^8	- - - - -	+ - - - -	PASS
Proteus vulgaris NCTC 4635				
Day 1	4.9×10^8	- - - - -	- - - - -	PASS
Day 2	8.8×10^8	- - - + -	- - - - -	PASS
Day 3	2.9×10^8	- - - - -	- - - - -	PASS
Escherischia coli NCTC 8196				
Day 1	6.9×10^8	- - - - -	- - - - -	PASS
Day 2	2.9×10^8	- - - - -	- - - - +	PASS
Day 3	2.7×10^8	+ - - - -	+ + - - -	PASS
Staphylococcus aureus NCTC 4163				
Day 1	9.0×10^8	- - - - -	- - + - +	PASS
Day 2	2.7×10^8	- - - - +	- - - - +	PASS
Day 3	5.8×10^8	- - + - -	- + - - -	PASS

The product marked "Tea Tree Oil 0166" was found to pass the T.G.A. test Opt B. All controls conformed to the requirements of the test system.

A THEORETICAL COMPARISON BETWEEN TEA TREE OIL AND OTHER ANTI-SEPTICS

(Extract from files of Museum of Applied Arts & Sciences, Sydney. 1974)

The following table is indicative only of the value of the Tea Tree Oil as an antiseptic product. To compile this table I have created a composite of the attributes referred to in the attached papers.

Product:	Gram positive [Staff aureus]	Gram negative [E. coli]	Acid fast bacillli	Bacterial spores	Fungicidal
Alcohols	Sensitive	Sensitive	Sensitive	Resistant	Moderate
Phenols	"	"	Non	"	Nil
Chlorine preps.	"	"	Mod. sensitive	Mod. sensitive	Nil
Iodine preps.	"	"	Sensitive	Resistant	Moderate
Aldehydes	"	"	"	Sensitive	Sensitive
Mercury preps.	"	Mod. sensitive	Resistant	Resistant	"
Chlorhexidine	"	" "	"	"	Resistant
Quat. Ammonium	"	" "	"	"	"
Tea Tree Oil	**Sensitive**	**Sensitive**	**Sensitive**	**Sensitive**	**Sensitive**

In addition to which Tea tree comes closest to fullfilling all 8 of Professor Anderson's properties for an ideal skin disinfectant. Taking his 8 attributes in order, Tea Tree Oil–

1. Has a rapid bacteriocidal action, occurring against a wide range of organisms, with good persistance, and with the added attribute of a high degree of absorption into the derma.
2. Possesses marked cleaning properties noted in the clerical literature repeatedly.
3. Is not easily contaminated.
4. Does not irritate the skin, is not poisonous, does not harm tissue cells, and has no significant side effects.
5. Is cosmetically very suitable, being colourless and of a pleasant, clean odour.
6. Is nearly neutral in Ph.
7. Is notably effective in the presence of organic detritus.
8. Is notably effective on fungi, and is used on viral complaints with success, though there is no available clinical work for this. It comes nearest therefore to being the ideal skin disinfectant.

This Clinical Data was performed and analyzed by E.M.L. consulting services of New Town, New South Wales, Australia.

Bibliography

Australian Journal of Pharmacy. Vol. 72, January, 1991.

Belaiche, P. "Treatment of Skin Infection with the Essential Oil of Melaleuca alternifolia." *Phylotherapie.* Vol. 15, 1985.

Belaiche, P. "Treatment of Vaginal Infections of Candida Albicans with the Essential Oil of Melaleuca alternifolia." *Phylotherapie.* Vol. 15, 1985.

Brown, Donald J., N.D. "Tea Tree Oil for Bacterial Vaginosis and Monilial Vulvovaginitis." *Townsend Letter for Doctors' Phytotherapy Review and Commentary.* May, 1991.

Goldsbrough, Robert E., F.C.S. "Ti-Tree Oil." *Manufacturing Chemist.* February, 1939, pp. 57-60.

The Medical Journal of Australia. Vol. 153, October 15, 1990.

Pena, E.O. "Melaleuca alternifolia Oil, Uses for Trichomonal Vaginitis and Other Vaginal Infections." *Obstetrics and Gynecology.* June, 1962.

Penfold, A.R., and Morrison, F.R. "Some Notes on the Essential Oil of M. alternifolia." *Australian Journal of Pharmacy.* March 30, 1930. *British Medical Journal, 1933.*

Australian Journal of Dentistry. August, 1930.

Shemesh, Alvin, M.D., and Mayo, William, Ph.D., *Family Practice Study.* May, 1991.

Tisserand, Robert. "Australian Tea Tree Oil." *Aromatherapy for Everyone.* April 28, 1988.

Walker, M. "Clinical Investigation of Australian Melaleuca alternifolia Oil for a Variety of Common Foot Problems." *Current Podiatry.* April, 1972.

Suggested Readings

Blumenthal, Mark. "Australian Tea Tree Oil." *The International Journal of Aromatherapy.* Vol. 1, No. 1, February, 1988.

Cusumano, Donna. "Australian Influence Making Inroads in the Marketplace." *Health Food Business Magazine.* February, 1988.

Tisserand, Robert. "Australian Tea Tree Oil." *The International Journal of Aromatherapy.* Vol. 1, No. 1, February, 1988.

Lee, Paul, Ph.D. "The Contemporary Herbal All About Tea Tree Oil From Australia." *Total Health Magazine,* 6001 Topanga Canyon Blvd., No. 3, Woodland Hills, CA 91367. October, 1988.

Blumenthal, Mark. "Herbs for Health, Tea Tree Oil." *Let's Live Magazine,* 444 N. Larchmont Blvd., Los Angeles, CA 90004. March, 1989.

Bunby, Paul. "Consumer Education Series: Tea Tree Oil." *Health Food Business,* Howmark Publishing Corp., 567 Morris Ave., Elizabeth, NJ 07208. July, 1989.

Reuben, Carolyn. *L.A. Weekly.* May 17-23, 1991.

Shimrod, Nimrod, N.D. "Body Care: Tea Tree Oil: Australian Gold." *Delicious Magazine,* New Hope Communicating Inc., 1301 Spruce Street, Boulder, CO 80302.

Day, Robb. "Alive, Focus on Nutrition #16, Australian Tea Tree Oil, The Essence of Excellence." This four-page report can be ordered by writing to *Alive, Focus on Nutrition,* Box 80055, Burnaby, B.C. V5H345 Canada.

Up and Coming Articles

Alive Magazine. July, August 1991 issue.

Rodale Press. *The Prevention How-To Dictionary of Healing Remedies and Techniques.* Early 1991 publication date.

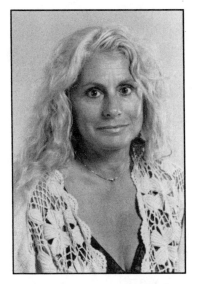

photo by Ray Szeflin

Cynthia Olsen lives her interest in health, healing and balance. Awareness of the unique healing properties of Tea Tree Oil led to this, her second book on the subject. This sharing is a continuing part of her balance of body, mind and spirit.

For additional books and information please write to:

Kali Press
P. O. Box 17628
Fountain Hills, Arizona 85269

This book printed on 100% recycled paper.